Read a Bit! Talk a Bit! is a series of reading activity books intended for people with dementia and Alzheimer's disease. The books start with a short article or story for the participants to read, followed by a number of questions for the facilitator to ask. These questions are formulated to engage the participants in conversation and to encourage personal and meaningful reminiscences to flow.

All the reading pages are in large type, 44 pt, and the text is only on one page per spread in order to help the individual to concentrate on the text and to minimize the constraints of visual impairment.

Memories recalled from earlier in life are often very therapeutic for people with dementia. They provide opportunities for positive and meaningful engagement with the past. Remembering increases self esteem and a feeling of positive worth as the participants recall personal experiences

These fifteen books successfully achieve this thanks to the range of familiar topics and questions to prompt and encourage discussions.

Mary Morris is a diversional therapist and Gunilla Denton Cook is the author of the acclaimed book Lost Words. Drawing on their knowledge and experience they have collaborated on this series of activity books.

I0424707

Read a Bit! Talk a Bit!
Titles available

At the Movies	**Safety pin**
Cake	**Sandwich**
Chickens	**Scissors**
Garden	**Soup**
Lawnmower	**Stamps**
Money	**Teddy Bear**
Pencil	**Telephone**
Perfume	

Published by:
Denton Cook Pty Ltd
15 Elabana Cr.
Castle Hill NSW 2154
Australia

Phone +61 2 9651 3558
Fax   +61 2 9651 3007
dentoncook@bigpond.com
www.readabittalkabit.com

Gardens have been a source of great pleasure for mankind since the beginning of time.

Pass to next reader

1

People have cultivated plants for food and for the pure enjoyment of beautiful flowers.

Pass to next reader

2

Garden written by Gunilla Denton Cook and Mary Morris.
©2010 Denton Cook Pty Ltd

Gardening is hard work. Today there are plenty of tools and machinery to help us do some of the tasks.

Pass to next reader

3

In spite of this, keen gardeners still insist on doing the work by hand. The hard work is part of the pleasure.

Pass to next reader

4

Garden written by Gunilla Denton Cook and Mary Morris.
©2010 Denton Cook Pty Ltd

There is a lot to be done. The soil has to be tended, weeds have to be removed and plants have to be cared for.

Garden written by Gunilla Denton Cook and Mary Morris.
©2010 Denton Cook Pty Ltd

The soil has to be prepared for the specific plants that will go into the area. Different plants have different needs to grow and show off the best possible display of color.

Pass to next reader

Garden written by Gunilla Denton Cook and Mary Morris.
©2010 Denton Cook Pty Ltd

Every gardener has his or her own passion. Some prefer to grow vegetables and others prefer to beautify their gardens with decorative plants.

7

Garden written by Gunilla Denton Cook and Mary Morris.
©2010 Denton Cook Pty Ltd

Local garden societies sometimes have competitions for best display or biggest vegetable grown.

Pass to next reader

8

Garden written by Gunilla Denton Cook and Mary Morris.
©2010 Denton Cook Pty Ltd

Most plants prefer a well drained organic soil. To achieve this takes a lot of manual labor.

Garden written by Gunilla Denton Cook and Mary Morris.
©2010 Denton Cook Pty Ltd

Compost is a good friend of all gardeners, but also requires constant attention to be the optimum additive for the garden.

Pass to next reader

10

Garden written by Gunilla Denton Cook and Mary Morris.
©2010 Denton Cook Pty Ltd

Many look on gardening as a relaxing activity and most would agree that a well-tended and beautifully designed garden is well worth the effort.

Pass to group leader

11

Garden written by Gunilla Denton Cook and Mary Morris.
©2010 Denton Cook Pty Ltd

Questions

1. Can you name a plant or a flower for every letter of the alphabet?

A   Amaryllis, aster, apricot...
B   Begonia, bougainvillea...
C   Cyclamen, cactus...
D   Daisy, daffodil...
E   Edelweiss...
F   Frangipani...
G   Gladiolus...
H   Hibiscus...
I   Iris...
J   Jasmine...
K   Kangaroo Paw...
L   Lily...
M   Magnolia...
N   Narcissus...
O   Orchid...
P   Philodendron...
Q   Quince...
R   Rose...
S   Sunflower...
T   Tulip...
U   Ulex...
V   Violet...
W   Wisteria...
X   Xanthorrhiza apiifolia...
Y   Yucca palm...
Z   Zinnia...

Garden written by Gunilla Denton Cook and Mary Morris.
©2010 Denton Cook Pty Ltd

2.   What is your favorite flower called?

3.   Have you ever succeeded with tulips?
     What is your secret?

4.   Why are some hydrangeas pink and others
     blue?

5.   Do you have a garden or potted plants that
     you tend?

6.   What kinds of tools do you use to weed with?

7.   What is your favorite activity in the garden?

8.   What kinds of plants are the easiest to
     grow?

9.   What is your favorite edible plant?

10. What can you do when your soil is heavy in
     clay?

11. What kind of fertilizer did you prefer to use
     in your garden? Blood and bone, compost,
     horse or chicken manure?

 Garden written by Gunilla Denton Cook and Mary Morris.
©2010 Denton Cook Pty Ltd

12. Fruit and vegetables always taste better when you grow them yourself. What did you grow for the family?

13. What vegetables did you have most success with and what did you do with any excess you may have had?

14. Insects can be both good and bad in the garden. What are some insects that you may find in a garden?

15. Can you name any insects that are good for the garden?

16. Who did the pruning in your garden? Was he, or she, a light or excessive pruner?

17. Where did you have your compost heap? What did you put on it?

18. Did you ever enter a gardening competition? Did you win?

19. How did you get new plants for your garden? (Seeds, seedlings, nursery, cuttings, grafting, swapping or stealing?)

Garden written by Gunilla Denton Cook and Mary Morris.
©2010 Denton Cook Pty Ltd

20. What sort of protective gear and equipment do you need for gardening?

21. Where do you keep your gardening equipment and how do you maintain it?

22. What other creatures shared your garden?

23. Did you grow up with lots of birds in the garden? What was it that attracted them to your garden?

Garden written by Gunilla Denton Cook and Mary Morris.
©2010 Denton Cook Pty Ltd